# NEUROPATHY DIET COOKBOOK FOR BEGINNERS

## HEALTHY NERVE-FRIENDLY RECIPES TO RELIEF PAIN, RESTORE SENSATION AND MANAGE WEAKNESS

**KAREN EDMONDS**

TABLE OF CONTENT

# INTRODUCTION

Welcome to the realm of nutrition-based neuropathy management! If you or a loved one suffer from neuropathy, a nerve-related ailment, this Neuropathy Diet Cookbook for Beginners can help make your journey more tasty and easy.

Neuropathy is more than just a medical word; it is a daily struggle for many. Numbness, tingling, and pain in the extremities can disrupt your life, but what you eat has a significant influence on how you feel. This cookbook is specifically developed for novices, offering a helpful approach to understanding neuropathy and adopting a nerve-healthy diet.

In this cookbook, we simplify difficult topics into manageable stages. Discover the link between neuropathy and your regular diet, as well as why certain foods might be beneficial. We will walk you through the basics, from identifying the many forms of neuropathy to consulting with healthcare providers and creating attainable dietary objectives.

Explore a selection of neuropathy-friendly dishes for breakfast, lunch, supper, snacks, and desserts. From nutrient-dense smoothies to one-pot marvels, these dishes prioritise antioxidants, omega-3 fatty acids, and low glycaemic index components.

However, it is not just about the recipes. We offer practical advice on diet planning, lifestyle adjustments, and commonly asked questions to help you along your neuropathy journey. Let us go on this cooking trip together, choosing delicious choices that feed both your body and your spirit. Here is to a neuropathy-friendly cookbook that provides joy to your kitchen and calms your nerves!

# CHAPTER 1

## What is Neuropathy?

Neuropathy, also known as peripheral neuropathy, is a disorder that affects the peripheral nerves—the network of nerves that surrounds the brain and spinal cord. These nerves are responsible for sending messages between the body and the central nervous system, allowing you to sense feelings and move your muscles. When these nerves are injured or malfunctioning, it can cause a variety of symptoms referred to as neuropathy.

Diabetes, infections, severe traumas, autoimmune illnesses, and toxic exposure are all potential causes of neuropathy. Numbness, tingling, discomfort, and weakness are common symptoms that begin in the hands or feet and progress to other areas.

**Types of Neuropathy**

- *Peripheral neuropathy:*

The most prevalent form, which affects the peripheral nerves of the body.

Numbness, tingling, and discomfort are common symptoms, which are commonly distributed "glove and stocking" style.

- *Diabetic neuropathy:*

Long-term diabetes causes a unique kind of peripheral neuropathy.

It mostly affects the nerves in the feet and legs, resulting in sensory loss and discomfort.

- *Autonomic Neuropathy:*

Affecting the nerves that regulate involuntary body activities including heart rate, digestion, and blood pressure.

Symptoms may include changes in heart rate, blood pressure, and gastrointestinal difficulties.

- *Focal neuropathy:*

Affected a single nerve or group of nerves, resulting in abrupt paralysis or discomfort.

Commonly related with nerve damage or compression.

* *Hereditary neuropathy:*

Caused by genetic mutations that alter nerve structure and function.

This category includes conditions such as Charcot-Marie-Tooth disease.

Understanding the precise form of neuropathy is critical for devising an effective treatment approach. Management frequently include treating the underlying cause, relieving symptoms, and making lifestyle changes, such as diet and exercise, to improve nerve health.

## How This Cookbook Can Help

This cookbook is more than simply a collection of dishes. It is a guide that will help you manage neuropathy via mindful eating. This is how it can make a difference.

***Education and awareness:***

Gain a thorough grasp of the relationship between neuropathy and food.

Learn about the important nutrients that promote nerve health and how particular foods might help relieve symptoms.

***Practical Tips for Beginners:***

Designed exclusively for novices, with step-by-step instructions and advice.

Make more educated decisions by learning about meal planning, grocery shopping, and altering classic recipes.

***Delicious and nutrient-dense recipes:***

Enjoy a selection of simple dishes with neuropathy-friendly ingredients.

Discover delicious meals for breakfast, lunch, supper, snacks, and desserts that focus on vital nutrients.

***Focus on Nerve-Boosting Elements:***

Antioxidants, omega-3 fatty acids, and meals with a low glycaemic index are all proven to improve nerve health.

Explore dishes that are not only delicious but also beneficial to your overall health.

***Meal Plan for Success:***

Practical meal plans that help you organise your eating habits.

You may easily incorporate these ideas into your daily life, creating stability and excellent results.

# Understanding Neuropathy and Diet.

Learn about the many types of neuropathy, including peripheral neuropathy and diabetic neuropathy.

Understand how each kind may necessitate certain nutritional concerns.

***Effect of Diet on Neuropathy Symptoms:***

Investigate how specific meals might alter neuropathy symptoms.

Learn how diet can help you manage pain, numbness, and other discomforts.

***Key Nutrients for Nerve Health:***

Learn about the essential nutrients that promote nerve function and healing.

Understand how including these nutrients into your diet might help with general nerve health.

***Consultation with Health Professionals:***

Emphasising the value of getting expert help for tailored recommendations.

Understand how healthcare specialists may help you adapt dietary advice based on your specific needs.

This cookbook is your guide to navigating the realm of neuropathy and food, giving both knowledge and practical tools for making beneficial changes in your everyday life.

# CHAPTER 2

## Impact of Diet on Neuropathy Symptoms

Diet has a big impact on neuropathy symptoms, and adopting smart dietary choices can help to manage and alleviate suffering. Here is how your food affects neuropathy symptoms:

*Inflammation reduction:*

Certain meals, particularly those strong in antioxidants, can help decrease inflammation. Chronic inflammation is associated with nerve injury and increased neuropathic pain.

*Blood Sugar Control:*

It is critical for people with diabetic neuropathy to keep their blood sugar constant. A low-glycemic index diet helps minimise blood sugar spikes and crashes, which reduces the risk of nerve damage.

### *Nerve Repair and Regeneration:*

Nutrient-dense diets give the necessary building blocks for nerve healing and regeneration. A well-balanced diet promotes the general health of nerve cells.

### *Weight Management:*

Maintaining a healthy weight helps to relieve strain on nerves, especially in disorders like peripheral neuropathy. A diet rich in full, nutrient-dense foods can help with weight management.

### *Enhanced Circulation:*

Certain nutrients, such as those found in diets high in omega-3 fatty acids, (found in fatty fish, flaxseeds, and walnuts) improve blood circulation. Improved circulation is essential for supplying nutrients to nerve cells.

### *Minimization of Neurotoxins:*

Certain chemicals can have neurotoxic properties. A diet rich in whole, unprocessed foods can help to reduce exposure to potentially harmful neurotoxins.

***Preventing Nutrient Deficiencies***:

B vitamins (B1, B6, and B12) are essential for nerve health. A well-balanced diet ensures that you get these important nutrients, preventing shortages that might worsen neuropathic symptoms.

***Balancing macronutrients:***

It is critical to maintain an appropriate carbohydrate, protein, and fat ratio. This helps to offer long-lasting energy, regulate blood sugar levels, and support general physiological activities.

***Hydration for overall wellness:***

Staying hydrated is critical for overall health, including nerve function. Water assists with biological processes, digestion, and toxin elimination.

***Individualised Dietary Approaches:***

Each individual's neuropathy experience is unique. Tailoring your diet to your unique requirements, tastes, and any underlying conditions results in a more personalised and effective symptom management strategy.

## Key Nutrients for Nerve Health

### B Vitamins:

Vitamins B1 (thiamine), B6 (pyridoxine), and B12 (cobalamin) are especially important for nerve health. Found in whole grains, nuts, seeds, and lean meats.

### Omega 3 Fatty Acids:

Supportive to nerve cell membranes and overall nerve function. Fatty fish (such as salmon and mackerel), flaxseeds, and walnuts are all good sources.

### Antioxidants:

Reduce oxidative stress and inflammation. Colourful fruits and vegetables include berries, spinach, and kale.

### Vitamin D:

Sunlight, fortified meals, and fatty seafood like salmon are all sources of this essential nutrient for nerve health.

### *Calcium and magnesium:*

Play a part in nerve transmission and muscle contraction. Dairy products, leafy greens, and nuts are excellent sources.

### *Alpha Lipoic Acid:*

Acts as a potent antioxidant and may alleviate neuropathic symptoms. Found in spinach, broccoli, and yeast.

### *Iron:*

Supports proper blood circulation and nerve oxygenation. Found in lean meats, beans, and dark leafy greens.

### Neuropathy-Friendly Foods

### *Fruits:*

Berries (including blueberries, strawberries, and raspberries) are high in antioxidants.

Citrus fruits (oranges, lemons) contain vitamin C, which aids immunological function.

### *Vegetables:*

Leafy greens (spinach and kale) are rich in antioxidants and vitamins.

Bell peppers contain both vitamin B6 and antioxidants.

### *Whole grains:*

Quinoa, brown rice, and oats are rich in complex carbs and vital elements including B vitamins.

### *Lean proteins:*

Skinless poultry, fish, tofu, and lentils provide protein without excessive saturated fats.

### *Fatty Fish:*

Salmon, mackerel, and sardines contain omega-3 fatty acids, which promote nerve function.

### *Nuts and seeds:*

Almonds, walnuts, and flax seeds are high in vitamin E and omega-3 fatty acids.

***Low-glycaemic index foods:***

Sweet potatoes, lentils, and healthy grains can help control blood sugar levels.

***Dairy or Dairy Alternative:***

Greek yoghurt, fortified almond milk, and cheese include calcium and vitamin D.

***Avocado:***

Avocado is high in healthful fats and vitamin E, which promote nerve health.

***Dark chocolate:***

In moderation, dark chocolate with a high cocoa content contains antioxidants.

***Herbs and spices:***

Turmeric, ginger, and cinnamon contain anti-inflammatory effects.

***Green Tea:***

Contains antioxidants and may have neuroprotective properties.

***Broccoli with cauliflower:***

Rich in fibre, vitamins, and antioxidants.

***Eggs:***

Provide B vitamins, especially B12, which is necessary for nerve function.

***Water:***

Staying hydrated is essential for good health and neurological function.

***Chia Seed:***

Rich in omega-3 fatty acids and fibre.

Understanding the relationship between food and neuropathy symptoms, as well as including these critical nutrients into your meals, will help you manage and improve your nerve health. Always seek personalised advice from healthcare specialists based on your individual medical situation.

# CHAPTER 3: RECIPES FOR BREAKFAST

## Nutrient-Packed Smoothies

**Ingredients:**

- 1 cup of mixed berries (blueberries, strawberries, raspberries)
- 1 average-sized banana, frozen
- 1 cup of leafy greens (spinach or kale)
- 1/2 cup of Greek yogurt (unsweetened)
- 1 tablespoon of chia seeds
- 1/2 cup of almond milk (unsweetened)
- 1/2 teaspoon of turmeric powder
- 1/2 teaspoon of freshly grated ginger
- 1 tablespoon of honey or maple syrup (optional for sweetness)
- Ice cubes (optional for thickness)

**Preparation:**

*Wash and Get ready the Ingredients:*

- Rinse the berries and leafy greens very well.

- Prior to using the banana, peel and freeze it.
- Measure the chia seeds and almond milk.

*Blend:*

- Blend the mixed berries, frozen banana, leafy greens, Greek yoghurt, chia seeds, almond milk, turmeric powder, and grated ginger.
- If you like it sweeter, add more honey or maple syrup.
- Blend at high speeds until smooth and creamy.

*Adjust consistency:*

- If your smoothie is too thick, add additional almond milk. If it is too thin, add ice cubes or more frozen fruit.

*Serve:*

- Pour your smoothie into a glass.

Garnish with chia seeds or a slice of fresh fruit, if preferred.

**Nutritional Value per Serving:**

Calories: Approximately 250-300 kcal

Protein: 10-15g

Fibre: 8-10g

Healthy Fats: 8-10g

Vitamins and Minerals: Rich in vitamin C, vitamin K, potassium, and antioxidants from berries and leafy greens.

Omega-3 Fatty Acids: Provided by chia seeds for nerve health.

Probiotics: Greek yogurt contributes to gut health.

Anti-Inflammatory Compounds: Turmeric and ginger add anti-inflammatory benefits.

# Notes

# Your

# Observation

# Whole Grain Breakfast Burrito

**Ingredients:**

- Whole wheat tortilla
- Scrambled eggs
- Black beans, cooked
- Salsa (homemade or store-bought)
- Avocado slices
- Shredded cheese (optional)
- Fresh cilantro, chopped (optional)
- Greek yogurt or low-fat sour cream (optional)
- Lime wedges for garnish

**Preparation:**

*Get ready the Scrambled Eggs:*

- In a bowl, whisk together the eggs and fry in a non-stick skillet until frothy.

*Warm tortillas:*

- Place the whole wheat tortilla on a hot griddle or pan and cook for a few seconds on each side until warmed.

*Assemble the Burrito:*

- Place the warmed tortilla on a flat surface.
- Spoon the scrambled eggs into the centre of the tortilla.

*Add black beans:*

- Spoon the cooked black beans over the scrambled eggs.

*Top with salsa:*

- For more flavour, add a big scoop of salsa. Adjust the quantity to suit your spice preferences.

*Include avocado slices:*

- Spread slices of ripe avocado over the remaining ingredients.

*Optional cheese:*

- Sprinkle with shredded cheese if desired. Choose a low- or reduced-fat variety.

*Optional: Fresh Cilantro*

- Add chopped fresh cilantro for a blast of herbaceous flavour.

*Fold & Roll:*

- Carefully fold the tortilla's sides in, then roll it up from the bottom to form a burrito.

*Serve with Greek yoghurt or sour cream:*

- Serve with a dollop of Greek yoghurt or low-fat sour cream on the side for a creamy finish.

*Garnish with lime:*

- Garnish with lime wedges for a citrus kick.

**Nutritional Value per Serving (Approximate):**

Calories: 350-400 kcal

Protein: Around 15-20g

Carbohydrates: About 35-40g

Dietary Fibre: 8-10g

Fats: 18-22g (Varies based on avocado and cheese use)

Saturated Fat: 4-6g (Varies based on cheese use)

Cholesterol: 200-250mg (Mainly from eggs)

Sodium: 600-700mg (Varies based on salsa and cheese)

Potassium: 500-600mg

Calcium: 150-200mg (Varies based on cheese use)

# Notes

# Your

# Observation

# Sweet Potato and Kale Hash with Fried Eggs

## Ingredients:

- Sweet potatoes, diced
- Kale leaves, chopped
- Red onion, finely sliced
- Eggs
- Olive oil or cooking spray
- Salt and pepper to taste
- Paprika (optional, for seasoning)

## Preparation:

*Prepare Vegetables:*

- Dice the sweet potatoes into tiny pieces.
- Chop the kale leaves and thinly slice the red onion.

*Sauté vegetables:*

- In a skillet set over medium heat, heat the olive oil or cooking spray.
- Add the cubed sweet potatoes and sauté until softened.

- Sauté the chopped greens and sliced red onion until they are soft.

*Season with spices:*

- To enhance flavour, season the mixture with salt, pepper, and (if desired) paprika.

*Create wells for eggs:*

- Make little wells or indentations in the hash using a spoon.

*Add eggs:*

- Crack eggs into each well of the hash.

*Cover and cook:*

- Cover the skillet and simmer until the eggs are cooked to your preference. For runny yolks, this might take a few minutes.

*Serve:*

- Carefully spoon out parts of the sweet potato and kale hash, topped with a fried egg.

*Season to taste:*

- If preferred, season with extra salt, pepper, or paprika.

**Nutritional Value per Serving (Approximate):**

Calories: 300-350 kcal

Protein: Around 12-15g

Carbohydrates: About 30-35g

Dietary Fibre: 5-8g

Fats: 15-18g

Saturated Fat: 3-4g

Cholesterol: 185-220mg

Sodium: 450-550mg

Potassium: 650-800mg

Vitamin A: 300-400% of daily recommended intake (mainly from sweet potatoes and kale)

Vitamin C: 50-70% of daily recommended intake (mainly from sweet potatoes)

Calcium: 10-15% of daily recommended intake

Iron: 15-20% of daily recommended intake

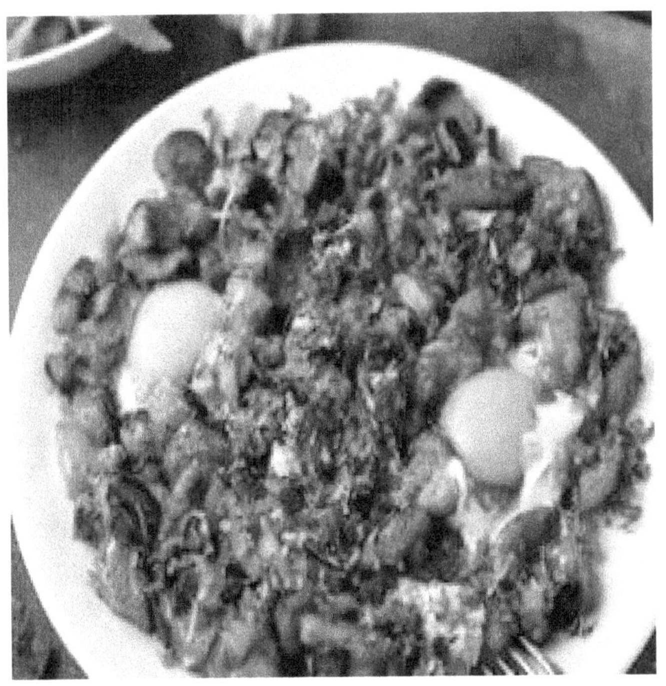

# Notes

# Your

# Observation

**Ingredients:**

- 3 big eggs
- 1/2 bell pepper (any color), chopped
- 1/2 onion, finely chopped
- 1 small tomato, chopped
- Handful of spinach leaves, chopped
- 1/4 cup of feta cheese, crumbled (optional)
- 1 tablespoon of olive oil
- Salt and pepper to taste
- Fresh herbs (such as parsley or chives) for garnish

**Preparation:**

- Dice the bell pepper, onion, tomato, and spinach.

*Whisk eggs:*

- Whisk the eggs until thoroughly blended in a mixing bowl. Season with salt and pepper.

*Sauté vegetables:*

- In a non-stick skillet, heat olive oil over medium heat.
- Add diced bell pepper and minced onion. Sauté until soft.

*Add tomato and spinach:*

- Add the diced tomatoes to the skillet. Stir until the tomatoes have released their juices.
- Add the chopped spinach and simmer until wilted.

*Pour eggs:*

- Pour the whisked eggs equally over the sautéed veggies.

*Cook the omelette:*

- Allow the eggs to set slightly around the edges. Use a spatula to raise the edges, allowing the raw eggs to flow to them.

*Optional Feta Cheese:*

- Sprinkle crumbled feta cheese over one side of the omelette.

*Fold and serve:*

- When the eggs are mostly set but still runny on top, use the spatula to fold the omelette in half.
- Cook for another minute, or until the cheese melts and the eggs are well cooked.

*Garnish and serve:*

- Slide the omelette to a plate. Garnish with fresh herbs and more salt and pepper if desired.
- Serve hot, and enjoy!

**Nutritional Values (Approximate):**

Calories: 250-300 kcal

Protein: 18g

Fat: 18g

Saturated Fat: 5g

Carbohydrates: 8g

Fibre: 2g

Cholesterol: 435mg

Sodium: 400mg

# Notes

# Your

# Observation

# Whole Grain Toast with Avocado

**Ingredients:**

- 2 pieces of whole grain bread
- 1 ripe avocado
- Cherry tomatoes, sliced (optional)
- Salt and pepper to taste
- Red pepper flakes (optional)
- Lemon juice (optional)

**Preparation:**

*Toast the Bread:*

- Toast two pieces of whole grain bread to the desired crispiness.

*Prepare the Avocado:*

- While the bread is toasting, split the avocado in half, remove the pit, and scoop out the meat into a dish.

*Mash the avocados:*

- Mash the avocado in the bowl with a fork until it is as smooth as you like.

*Season the avocado:*

- Add salt and pepper to the mashed avocado. For an extra kick, sprinkle with red pepper flakes.

*Spread avocado on toast:*

- Spread the mashed avocado equally on each slice of toasted whole grain bread.

*Optional toppings:*

- Garnish with sliced cherry tomatoes for a punch of brightness. Drizzle with lemon juice to enhance flavour.

*Serve and enjoy:*

- Transfer the avocado toast to a platter and serve immediately.

**Nutritional Values (Approximate):**

Calories: 250-300 kcal

Protein: 7g

Fat: 15g

Saturated Fat: 2g

Carbohydrates: 28g

Fibre: 10g

Cholesterol: 0mg

Sodium: 250mg

# Notes

# Your

# Observation

# CHAPTER 4: LUNCH AND DINNER RECIPES

## Grilled Chicken Breast

**Ingredients:**

- 4 boneless, skinless chicken breasts
- 2 tablespoons of olive oil
- 1 teaspoon of garlic powder
- 1 teaspoon of paprika
- Salt and pepper to taste

**Preparation:**

- Preheat the grill or grill pan to medium-high heat.
- Combine the olive oil, garlic powder, paprika, salt, and pepper to make a marinade in a small bowl.
- Pat the chicken breasts dry and then brush with the marinade on both sides.
- Cook the chicken breasts on the prepared grill for 6-8 minutes each side, or until the internal temperature reaches

165°F (74°C) and the centre is no longer pink.

*Serve:*

- Let the chicken rest for a few minutes before serving.

**Nutritional Values (Per 3 oz cooked):**

Calories: 165 kcal

Protein: 31g

Fat: 3.6g

Saturated Fat: 0.9g

Carbohydrates: 0g

Fibre: 0g

Cholesterol: 85mg

Sodium: 75mg

# Notes

# Your

# Observation

# Baked Salmon

**Ingredients:**

- 4 salmon fillets
- 2 tablespoons of lemon juice
- 1 tablespoon of olive oil
- 2 cloves of minced garlic
- 1 teaspoon of dried dill
- Salt and pepper to taste

**Preparation:**

- Preheat the oven to 400 °F (200 °C).
- Place the salmon fillets on a baking sheet.
- In a small bowl, combine the lemon juice, olive oil, minced garlic, dried dill, salt, and pepper.
- Brush the mixture on the fish.
- Bake for 12-15 minutes, or until salmon flakes readily with a fork.
- Broil for a further 2-3 minutes to achieve a golden crust on top. (Optional)

- Then serve and enjoy

**Nutritional Values (Per 3 oz cooked):**

Calories: 180 kcal

Protein: 22g

Fat: 9g

Saturated Fat: 1.5g

Carbohydrates: 0g

Fiber: 0g

Cholesterol: 55mg

Sodium: 65mg

## Notes

## Your

## Observation

# Chicken and Vegetable Quinoa Bowl

**Ingredients:**

- Boneless, skinless chicken breasts
- Quinoa
- Mixed vegetables (bell peppers, zucchini, carrots)
- Chicken broth
- Olive oil
- Garlic, minced
- Paprika, cumin, salt, and pepper for seasoning

**Preparation:**

- Sauté chicken in olive oil until brown. Remove and place aside.
- In the same saucepan, sauté the garlic and vegetables.
- Combine the quinoa, chicken broth, and spices.
- Place the chicken on top, cover, and boil until the quinoa is cooked.
- Serve

**Nutritional Value (Approximate per Serving):**

Calories: 400-450 kcal

Protein: 30g

Carbohydrates: 40g

Fiber: 5g

Fat: 15g

# Notes

# Your

# Observation

## Ingredients:

- Chickpeas (canned or cooked)
- Spinach leaves
- Tomatoes, chooped (canned or fresh)
- Onion, diced
- Garlic, minced
- Vegetable broth
- Olive oil
- Cumin, coriander, salt, and pepper for seasoning

## Preparation:

- Sauté onion and garlic in olive oil until softened.
- Combine chickpeas, chopped tomatoes, and vegetable broth.
- Season with cumin, coriander, salt, and pepper.
- Stir in the spinach and cook until wilted.

- Serve

**Nutritional Value (Approximate per Serving):**

Calories: 300-350 kcal

Protein: 12g

Carbohydrates: 50g

Fiber: 12g

Fat: 8g

# Notes

# Your

# Observation

# Salmon and Quinoa Pilaf

**Ingredients:**

- Salmon fillets
- Quinoa
- Cherry tomatoes, halved
- Spinach leaves
- Chicken broth
- Lemon juice
- Dill, salt, and pepper for seasoning

**Preparation:**

- Season the salmon with lemon juice, dill, salt, and pepper.
- In a saucepan, sear the fish until well cooked.
- In the same saucepan, add the quinoa, chicken broth, cherry tomatoes, and spinach.
- Simmer until the quinoa is cooked and the vegetables are soft.
- Serve

**Nutritional Value (Approximate per Serving):**

Calories: 350-400 kcal

Protein: 25g

Carbohydrates: 30g

Fiber: 4g

Fat: 15g

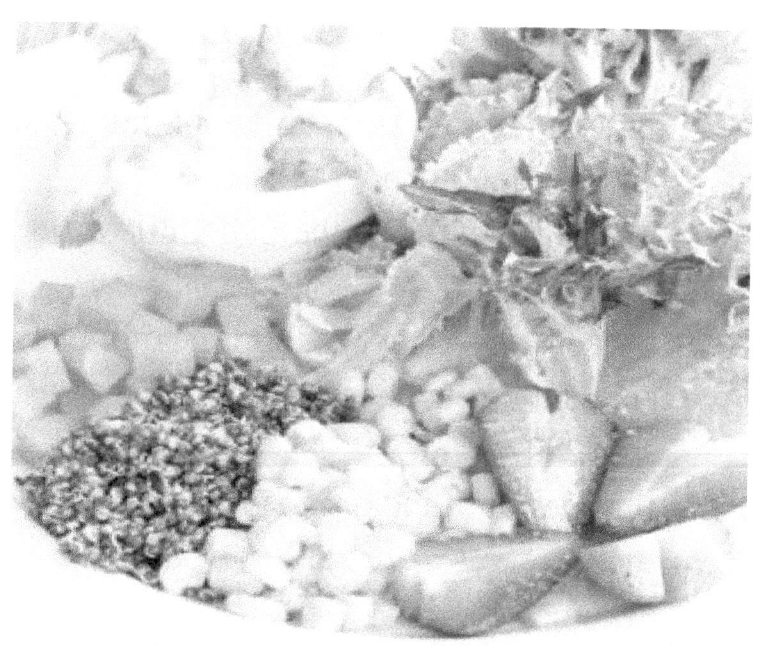

# Notes

# Your

# Observation

## Fibre-Rich Vegetable and Grain Bowl

**Ingredients:**

- 1 cup of Quinoa (rinsed)
- 1 cup of Broccoli florets
- 1 cup of Carrot (sliced)
- 1 cup of Bell peppers (diferent colours), (chopped)
- 2 cups of Spinach (chopped)
- 1 cup of Cherry tomatoes (halved)
- 2 tablespoons of Olive oil
- 2 cloves of minced Garlic
- 1 tablespoon of lemon juice
- Salt and pepper: to taste
- Optional toppings: Avocado slices, sesame seeds, or feta cheese.

**Preparation:**

- *Cook Quinoa*:

In a saucepan, mix quinoa and 2 cups water. Bring to a boil, then decrease heat, cover, and simmer for 15 minutes, or until the quinoa is cooked and the water has been absorbed.

- *Roast Vegetables*:

Preheat the oven to 400°F (200°C). Toss the broccoli, carrots, and bell peppers with olive oil, minced garlic, salt, and pepper. Roast in the oven for 20-25 minutes, or until veggies are soft.

- *Assemble bowl:*

In a serving bowl, mix together cooked quinoa, roasted veggies, spinach, and cherry tomatoes.

- *Dressing*:

Drizzle the bowl with lemon juice and an extra tablespoon olive oil. Toss the ingredients until uniformly coated.

Optional toppings include avocado slices, sesame seeds, and crumbled feta cheese for added flavour and texture.

**Nutritional Value (Approximate per Serving):**

Calories: 400

Protein: 12g

Fat: 15g

Saturated Fat: 2g

Monounsaturated Fat: 10g

Polyunsaturated Fat: 2g

Carbohydrates: 60g

Dietary Fiber: 12g

Sugars: 6g

# Notes

# Your

# Observation

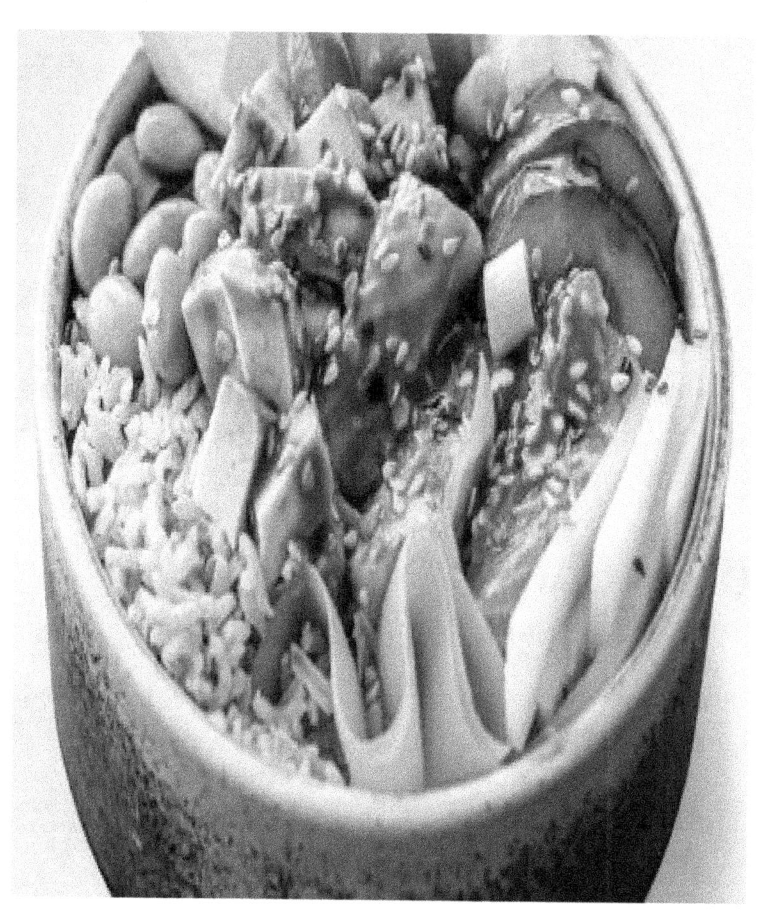

# CHAPTER 5: SNACKS AND APPETIZERS

## Almonds

**Ingredients:**

- Raw almonds

**Preparation:**

- Use sliced or chopped almonds as a topping for yogurt or salads.
- To make almond butter, mix almonds in a food processor until smooth.
- Enjoy almonds as a snack.

**Nutritional Value (per 1 oz serving):**

Calories: 160

Protein: 6g

Fat: 14g

Carbohydrates: 6g

Fibre: 3.5g

# Pistachios

**Ingredients:**

- Raw pistachios

**Preparation:**

- Eat pistachios as a snack.
- Add pistachios to trail mix or yogurt.
- Crush pistachios and use as a coating for chicken or fish.

**Nutritional Value (per 1 oz serving):**

Calories: 160

Protein: 6g

Fat: 14g

Carbohydrates: 8g

Fibre: 3g

# Chia Seeds

**Ingredients:**

Chia seeds

**Preparation:**

- To make chia pudding, mix chia seeds with yoghurt.
- Add chia seeds to smoothies or oatmeal.
- Make chia seed jam by mixing with fruit and allowing it to thicken.

**Nutritional Value (per 1 oz serving):**

Calories: 138

Protein: 5g

Fat: 9g

Carbohydrates: 12g

Fiber: 10g

# Notes

## Your

## Observation

# Apple Slices with Almond Butter

**Ingredients:**

- Apples, sliced
- Almond butter

**Preparation:**

- Spread almond butter on apple slices.
- Enjoy as a quick and filling snack.

**Nutritional Value (Approximate per Serving):**

Calories: 120

Protein: 2g

Fat: 7g

Saturated Fat: 0.5g

Monounsaturated Fat: 4.5g

Polyunsaturated Fat: 1g

Carbohydrates: 15g

Fibre: 3g

Sugars: 9g



# Berries and Greek Yogurt Parfait

**Ingredients:**

- Mixed berries (strawberries, blueberries, raspberries)
- Greek yogurt
- Honey (optional)

**Preparation:**

- Prepare by layering fruit and Greek yoghurt in a glass.
- Drizzle with honey if preferred.

**Nutritional Value (Approximate per Serving):**

Calories: 150

Protein: 12g

Fat: 2g

Saturated Fat: 1g

Trans Fat: 0g

Carbohydrates: 25g

Fiber: 4g

Sugars: 18g

## Watermelon Cubes with Feta and Mint

**Ingredients:**

- Watermelon, cubed
- Feta cheese, crumbled
- Fresh mint leaves

**Preparation:**

- Mix watermelon cubes and feta.
- Garnish with fresh mint.

**Nutritional Value (Approximate per Serving):**

Calories: 100

Protein: 3g

Fat: 5g

Saturated Fat: 3g

Trans Fat: 0g

Carbohydrates: 12g

Fiber: 1g

Sugars: 9g

## Banana and Peanut Butter Roll-Ups

**Ingredients:**

- Banana
- Whole-grain tortilla
- Peanut butter

**Preparation:**

- Spread peanut butter on a tortilla.
- Place a banana and wrap it up.

**Nutritional Value (Approximate per Serving):**

Calories: 200

Protein: 6g

Fat: 9g

Saturated Fat: 2g

Monounsaturated Fat: 4g

Polyunsaturated Fat: 2g

Carbohydrates: 28g

Fiber: 3g

Sugars: 14g

## Orange and Cottage Cheese Bowl

**Ingredients:**

- Orange segments
- Cottage cheese

**Preparation:**

- Add orange segments with cottage cheese.
- Mix well and enjoy.

**Nutritional Value (Approximate per Serving):**

Calories: 150

Protein: 13g

Fat: 3g

Saturated Fat: 2g

Trans Fat: 0g

Carbohydrates: 18g

Fiber: 3g

Sugars: 14g

# Notes




# Your

# Observation

**Ingredients:**

- Ripe avocados, mashed
- Diced tomatoes
- Red onion, finely chopped
- Garlic, minced
- Lime juice
- Fresh cilantro, chopped
- Salt and pepper to taste

**Preparation:**

- Combine mashed avocados, tomatoes, red onion, garlic, lime juice, and cilantro in a bowl.
- Season with salt and pepper. Mix very well and serve.

**Nutritional Value (Approximate per Serving):**

Calories: 120

Protein: 2g

Fat: 10g

Saturated Fat: 1.5g

Monounsaturated Fat: 7g

Polyunsaturated Fat: 1.5g

Carbohydrates: 8g

Fiber: 6g

Sugars: 1g

## Salsa Fresca

**Ingredients:**

- Tomatoes, chopped
- Red onion, thinly chopped
- Jalapeño, seeded and diced
- Fresh cilantro, chopped
- Lime juice
- Salt to taste

**Preparation:**

- Combine diced tomatoes, red onion, jalapeño, and cilantro in a bowl.
- Add lime juice and salt. Mix very well.

**Nutritional Value (Approximate per Serving):**

Calories: 15

Protein: 1g

Fat: 0g

Carbohydrates: 4g

Fibre: 1g

Sugars: 2g

## Hummus

**Ingredients:**

- Chickpeas (canned or cooked)
- Tahini
- Olive oil
- Garlic, minced
- Lemon juice
- Cumin, salt, and pepper to taste

**Preparation:**

- Blend chickpeas, tahini, olive oil, minced garlic, and lemon juice until smooth.
- Season with cumin, salt, and pepper.

**Nutritional Value (Approximate per Serving):**

Calories: 70

Protein: 3g

Fat: 5g

Saturated Fat: 0.5g

Monounsaturated Fat: 3g

Polyunsaturated Fat: 1g

Carbohydrates: 6g

Fiber: 2g

Sugars: 1g

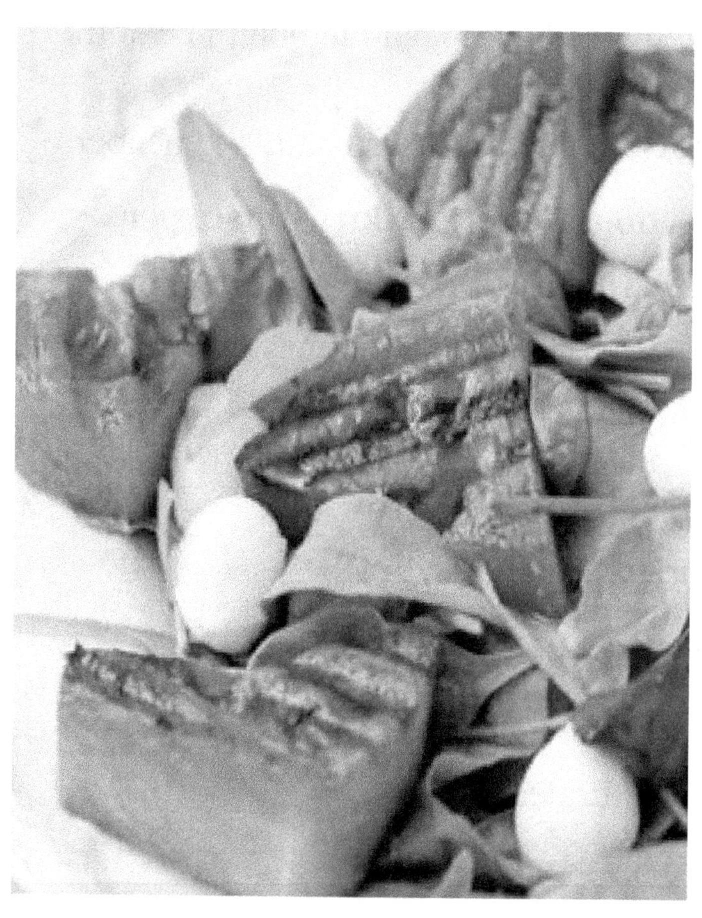

# CHAPTER 6: DESSERTS DELIGHT

## Stevia-Sweetened Chocolate Avocado Mousse

**Ingredients:**

- 2 ripe avocados
- 1/4 cup of unsweetened cocoa powder
- 1/4 cup of almond milk
- 1 teaspoon of vanilla extract
- Stevia to taste

**Preparation:**

- Prepare by blending avocados, chocolate powder, almond milk, and vanilla extract until creamy.
- Add stevia to create the desired sweetness.
- Chill before serving.

**Nutritional Value (Approximate per Serving):**

Calories: 150

Protein: 3g

Fat: 12g

Saturated Fat: 2g

Monounsaturated Fat: 8g

Polyunsaturated Fat: 1.5g

Carbohydrates: 10g

Fibre: 6g

Sugars: 1g

## Almond Flour Berry Crumble

**Ingredients:**

- 2 cups of mixed berries (strawberries, blueberries, raspberries)
- 1 cup of almond flour
- 1/4 cup of melted coconut oil
- Stevia or erythritol to taste
- Dash of cinnamon

**Preparation:**

- Combine berries in a baking dish.

- In a bowl, add almond flour, melted coconut oil, sweetener, and cinnamon.
- Crumble the mixture over the berries.
- Bake until the top is brown and the berries bubble.
- Then serve

**Nutritional Value (Approximate per Serving):**

Calories: 200

Protein: 4g

Fat: 15g

Saturated Fat: 7g

Monounsaturated Fat: 6g

Polyunsaturated Fat: 1g

Carbohydrates: 16g

Fibre: 6g

Sugars: 6g

# Sugar-Free Greek Yogurt Popsicles

**Ingredients:**

- 2 cups of Greek yogurt
- 1 cup of unsweetened almond milk
- Berries or sliced fruit
- Stevia or monk fruit sweetener to taste

**Preparation:**

- Combine Greek yoghurt, almond milk, and sweetener.
- Fill popsicle moulds with berries or other fruit.
- Freeze until solid.
- Serve

**Nutritional Value (Approximate per Serving):**

Calories: 80

Protein: 5g

Fat: 4g

Saturated Fat: 2g

Monounsaturated Fat: 1g

Polyunsaturated Fat: 0g

Carbohydrates: 7g

Fibre: 1g

Sugars: 4g

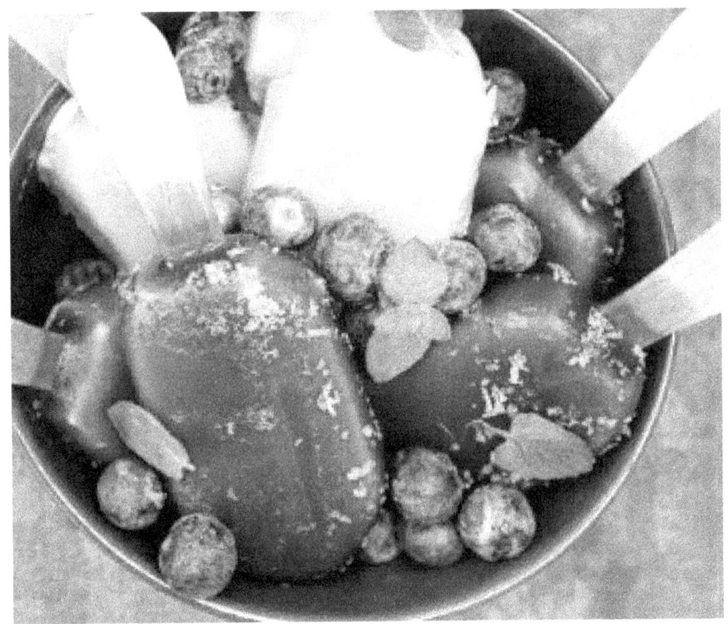

# Notes

# Your

# Observation

# Frozen Banana Bites

**Ingredients:**

- Bananas, sliced
- Dark chocolate, melted
- Chopped nuts or shredded coconut (optional for coating)

**Preparation:**

- Dip banana slices into melted dark chocolate.
- Coat with chopped nuts or shredded coconut if preferred.
- Place on a parchment-lined pan and freeze until firm.

**Nutritional Value (Approximate per Serving):**

Calories: 80

Protein: 1g

Fat: 4g

Saturated Fat: 2g

Monounsaturated Fat: 1g

Polyunsaturated Fat: 0.5g

Carbohydrates: 12g

Fibre: 2g

Sugars: 6g

## Watermelon Mint Salad

- **Ingredients:**
- Watermelon (cut in cubes)
- Fresh mint leaves, chopped
- Feta cheese, crumbled (optional)
- Balsamic glaze (optional)

**Preparation:**

- Combine watermelon cubes with chopped mint.
- If preferred, sprinkle with crumbled feta.
- Drizzle with balsamic glaze for added flavour.

**Nutritional Value (Approximate per Serving):**

Calories: 50

Protein: 1g

Fat: 1g

Saturated Fat: 0g

Monounsaturated Fat: 0g

Polyunsaturated Fat: 0g

Carbohydrates: 12g

Fibre: 1g

Sugars: 9g

## Mango Coconut Chia Pudding

**Ingredients:**

- Mango, blended
- Chia seeds
- Coconut milk
- Unsweetened shredded coconut (optional for topping)

**Preparation:**

- Combine blended mango, chia seeds, and coconut milk.
- Refrigerate until the chia pudding has set.
- If preferred, add some shredded coconut on top.

**Nutritional Value (Approximate per Serving):**

Calories: 160

Protein: 3g

Fat: 8g

Saturated Fat: 5g

Monounsaturated Fat: 1g

Polyunsaturated Fat: 1g

Carbohydrates: 20g

Fibre: 6g

Sugars: 12g

## Notes

## Your

## Observation

# Dark Chocolate-Dipped Strawberries

**Ingredients:**

- Fresh strawberries
- Dark chocolate (70% cocoa or more)
- Chopped nuts or shredded coconut (optional for coating)

**Preparation:**

- Melt dark chocolate in a heat-proof basin.
- Dip each strawberry in the melted chocolate.
- Place on a parchment-lined dish and top with nuts or shredded coconut, if preferred.
- Let the chocolate set.

# Dark Chocolate and Almond Clusters

**Ingredients:**

- Dark chocolate chips
- Almonds, whole or sliced
- Sea salt (optional for sprinkling)

**Preparation:**

- Melt dark chocolate in a microwave-safe bowl.
- Stir in almonds until well coated.
- Spoon clusters onto a parchment-lined tray.
- Sprinkle with sea salt if preferred and let them cool.

# Dark Chocolate Avocado Mousse

**Ingredients:**

- Ripe avocados

- Dark chocolate (70% cocoa or more), melted
- Unsweetened cocoa powder
- Maple syrup or honey for sweetness

**Preparation:**

- Blend ripe avocados **until** smooth.
- Add melted dark chocolate, cocoa powder, and sweeten to taste.
- Chill before serving.

## Chocolate-Covered Almond Stuffed Dates

**Ingredients:**

Medjool dates, pitted

Dark chocolate (70% cocoa or more)

Almonds, whole or almond butter

**Preparation:**

- Stuff each date with one whole almond or a little bit of almond butter.
- Dip the filled dates in melted dark chocolate.
- Allow the chocolate to set on a tray lined with parchment paper.

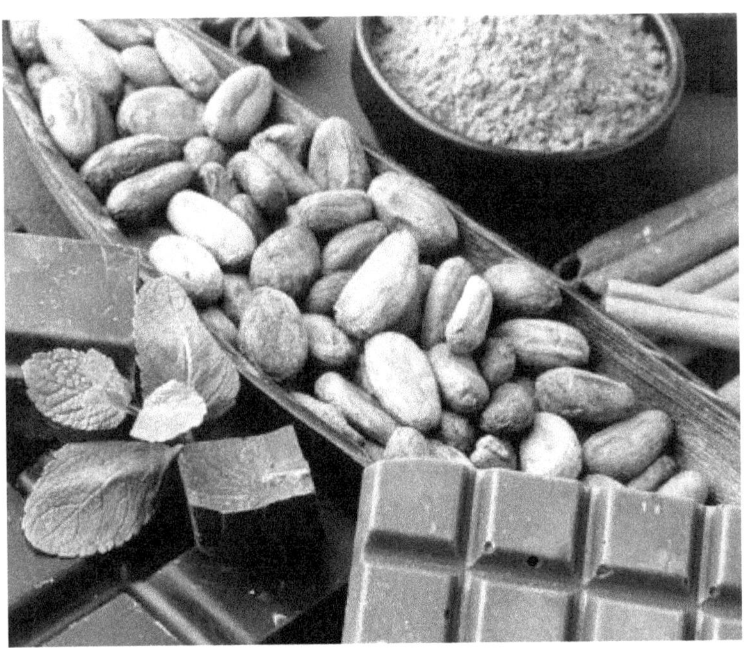

**Notes**

**Your**

**Observation**

# CHAPTER 7: BEVERAGES FOR NERVE HEALTH

## Turmeric Golden Milk

**Ingredients:**

- 1 cup of almond milk (or any milk of choice)
- 1/2 teaspoon of turmeric powder
- 1/4 teaspoon of cinnamon
- 1/4 teaspoon of ginger powder
- 1 teaspoon of honey (optional for sweetness)

**Preparation:**

- Heat almond milk in a saucepan.
- Combine turmeric, cinnamon, and ginger.
- Stir thoroughly and allow it boil for a few minutes.
- Honey can be added if desired. Strain, and enjoy.

**Benefits:**

Turmeric has anti-inflammatory properties.

Ginger supports digestive health.

## Berry Antioxidant Smoothie

**Ingredients:**

- 1/2 cup of mixed berries (blueberries, raspberries, strawberries)
- 1/2 banana
- 1 cup of spinach leaves
- 1/2 cup of Greek yogurt
- 1 cup of water or coconut water

**Preparation:**

- Mix berries, banana, spinach, Greek yoghurt, and water in a blender until smooth.
- Pour in a glass and enjoy.

**Benefits:**

Berries are rich in antioxidants.

Spinach provides essential vitamins.

## Green Tea with Lemon

**Ingredients:**

- 1 green tea bag
- 1 cup of hot water
- Slices of fresh lemon
- Honey (optional for sweetness)

**Preparation:**

- To prepare, steep a green tea bag in boiling water.
- If desired, combine lemon slices and honey.
- Stir and enjoy

**Benefits:**

Green tea contains antioxidants.

Lemon adds vitamin C for immune support.

## Ingredients:

- Thin slices of cucumber
- Fresh mint leaves
- 1 litre of water
- Ice cubes

## Preparation:

- Prepare by combining cucumber slices and mint leaves in a pitcher.
- Add water and chill for a few hours.
- Serve over ice.

## Benefits:

Cucumber provides hydration.

Mint aids digestion.

# Notes

# Your
# Observation

# Chamomile Lavender Tea

**Ingredients:**

- 1 chamomile tea bag
- 1 teaspoon of dried lavender buds
- Honey (optional for sweetness)

**Preparation:**

- Prepare by steeping the chamomile tea bag and dried lavender in boiling water.
- Allow it to steep for 5–7 minutes.
- Strain, add honey if desired, and serve.

**Health Benefits:**

Chamomile may promote relaxation.

Lavender is known for its calming properties.

# Peppermint Eucalyptus Infusion

**Ingredients:**

- 1 peppermint tea bag
- Fresh or dried eucalyptus leaves (1 teaspoon)
- Lemon wedge (optional)

**Preparation:**

- Steep the peppermint tea bag and eucalyptus leaves in boiling water.
- Allow it steep for 5-7 minutes.
- Add a lemon wedge for extra flavour if preferred.
- Strain and enjoy.

**Health Benefits:**

Peppermint supports digestion.

Eucalyptus may have respiratory benefits.

## Ginger Turmeric Herbal Tea

**Ingredients:**

- 1 tablespoon of Fresh ginger slices
- ½ teaspoon of Ground turmeric

- 1 herbal tea bag (e.g., lemongrass or ginger tea)
- Honey for sweetness (optional)

## Preparation:

- Boil fresh ginger slices in water.
- Combine ground turmeric and the herbal tea bag.
- Allow it to steep for 5-7 minutes.
- Strain, add honey if preferred, and enjoy.

## Health Benefits:

Ginger and turmeric have anti-inflammatory properties.

## Lemon Balm Mint Infusion

## Ingredients:

- 1 tablespoon of Fresh lemon balm leaves
- 1 tablespoon of Fresh mint leaves
- 1 green tea bag
- Lemon slice (optional)

**Preparation**:

- Steep lemon balm and mint leaves along with the green tea bag.
- Allow it to steep for 5-7 minutes.
- Add a lemon slice for freshness if preferred.
- Strain and enjoy.

**Health Benefits:**

Lemon balm may have calming effects.

Mint aids digestion.

Hibiscus Rosehip Tea

**Ingredients:**

1 tablespoon of dried hibiscus petals (1 tablespoon)

- 1 tablespoon of  dried rosehips (1 tablespoon)
- 1 hibiscus tea bag
- Agave syrup for sweetness (optional)

**Preparation:**

- Steep dried hibiscus petals, dried rosehips, and the hibiscus tea bag in hot water.
- Allow it to steep for 7-10 minutes.
- Add agave syrup for sweetness if preferred.
- Strain and enjoy.

**Health Benefits:**

Hibiscus may help lower blood pressure.

Rosehips are rich in vitamin C.

# Notes

# Your

# Observation

## HYDRATION TIPS FOR NEUROPATHY:

- ***Regular Water Intake:***

*Tip:* Drink water regularly throughout the day.

*Why:* Proper hydration promotes nerve function and general wellness.

- ***Enhance Water Flavour:***

*Tip:* Add natural flavours such as lemon, cucumber, or mint to make it more pleasant.

*Why*: Flavouring water might lead to greater consumption

- ***Limit Caffeine and Alcohol:***

*Tip:* Reduce caffeine beverages and alcoholic consumption.

*Why:* Caffeine and alcohol can cause dehydration; moderation is crucial.

- ***Monitor Electrolyte Levels:***

*Tip:* Eat electrolyte-rich meals like bananas, oranges, and leafy greens.

*Why:* Electrolytes are essential for nerve activity and fluid homeostasis

- ***Choose Hydrating Foods:***

*Tip*: Include water-rich foods like watermelon, cucumber, and celery in your diet.

*Why:* Hydrating meals increase total fluid consumption.

- ***Set Hydration Goals:***

*Tip*: Set daily hydration goals and track *intake with a water bottle.*

*Why*: Goals assist to maintain regular water drinking.

- ***Listen to Your Body:***

***Tip:*** Recognise thirst signs and drink water accordingly.

*Why:* Thirst is your body's natural indication that it needs to be re-hydrated.

- ***Stay Hydrated During Exercise:***

*Tip:* Remember to drink water before, during, and after physical activity.

*Why:* Exercise increases fluid requirements, and staying hydrated promotes overall health.

- ***Consult with Healthcare Professionals:***

*Tip*: Ask your healthcare team for personalised hydration recommendations.

*Why:* Neuropathy care may necessitate individualised counsel.

- ***Manage Underlying disorders:***

*Tip*: Treat any underlying disorders that may be causing neuropathy.

*Why:* Addressing the underlying reason can improve both symptoms and general health.

- ***Be Mindful of medications:***

*Tip*: Consult your healthcare practitioner if any drugs may affect your hydration levels.

*Why:* Some drugs can disrupt fluid balance.

- ***Warm Water Soaks:***

*Tip:* Try warm water soaks for hands or feet.

*Why:* Warm water can bring relief and induce relaxation.

- ***Avoid dehydrating elements:***

*Tip*: Limit exposure to elements that cause dehydration, such hot temperatures or frequent perspiration.

*Why:* Prevention is essential for staying hydrated.

- ***Hydrate Before Bed:***

*Tip*: Drink a small amount of water before bedtime.

*Why:* Adequate hydration supports overall bodily functions even during sleep.

- ***Monitor Fluid consumption:***

*Tip:* Use a hydration app or notebook to track daily fluid consumption.

*Why:* Tracking helps you achieve your hydration goals.

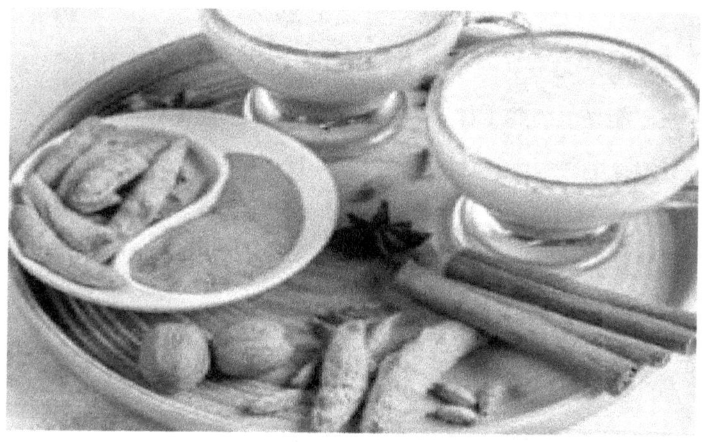

# CHAPTER 8: MEAL PLANNING TIPS

Meal planning is an essential part of eating a healthy, balanced diet. Here are some suggestions to help you make healthful and delicious meals:

- ***Set Realistic Goals:***

*Tip:* Determine your dietary goals, such as weight control, enhanced energy, or particular nutritional requirements.

*Why:* Setting specific goals provides focus and inspiration for your meal planning efforts.

- ***Make a Weekly Schedule:***

*Tip:* Plan your meals for the week, including breakfast, lunch, supper, and snacks.

*Why*: Having a defined strategy allows you to make better choices while decreasing the probability of last-minute harmful decisions.

- ***Eat a Variety of Nutrients:***

*Tip*: Include lean meats, whole grains, fruits, vegetables, and healthy fats in every meal.

*Why:* A diversified food diet promotes overall health and includes a variety of critical vitamins and minerals.

- ***Preparing Ingredients in Advance:***

*Tip:* Wash, cut, and portion vegetables, fruits, and meats ahead of time.

*Why:* Preparing food saves time on hectic days and makes it simpler to keep to your meal plan.

- ***Shop with a List:***

*Tip:* Plan your meals ahead of time and develop a grocery list.

*Why:* Shopping with a list keeps you focused, prevents impulse purchases, and ensures you have the supplies you need for your meals.

- ***Batch Cook and Freeze:***

*Tip*: Batch cook and freeze individual servings for future use.

*Why:* Batch cooking saves time, ensuring that there is always a healthy alternative accessible, and avoids food waste.

- ***Mind Portion Sizes:***

*Tip:* Be cautious of portion amounts to *prevent overeating.*

*Why*: Proper portion control promotes weight management and prevents excessive calorie consumption.

- ***Try fresh meals:***

*Tip:* Include fresh and fascinating meals in your food plan.

*Why:* Trying different recipes makes meals more exciting and exposes you to a wide range of flavours and cuisines.

- ***Balance Macronutrients:***

*Tip:* Try fresh meals: Tip: Include fresh and fascinating meals in your food plan.

*Why:* Trying different recipes makes meals more exciting and exposes you to a wide range of flavours and cuisines.

- ***Keep Hydrated:***

*Tip:* Include water in your meal plan to keep hydrated all day.

*Why:* Proper hydration improves digestion, nutrition absorption, and general health.

- ***Listen to Your Body:***

*Tip*: Pay attention to hunger and fullness signals.

*Why*: Eating when hungry and ending when full encourages intuitive eating and improves overall health.

- ***Plan for Special Occasions:***

*Tip:* Plan meals around forthcoming events or social gatherings.

*Why:* Planning for special events helps you to enjoy them while maintaining your overall healthy eating habits.

- **Be Flexible:**

*Tip:* Be open to changes in your eating plan.

*Why*: Flexibility enables you to respond to changing situations while maintaining a healthy connection with food.

- ***Seek Professional Guidance:***

*Tip:* Consult a Registered Dietitian or Nutritionist for Personalised Advice.

*Why*: Professionals can offer specialised advice based on your specific health requirements and goals.

- ***Practice Moderation:***

*Tip:* Enjoy indulgences in moderation instead than limiting particular meals.

*Why*: Moderation encourages a long-term approach to healthy eating and decreases the likelihood of feeling deprived.

## Lifestyle Changes for Neuropathy

- ***Maintaining Healthy Blood Sugar Levels:***

*Why?* Blood sugar levels must be managed carefully for people suffering from diabetes-related neuropathy.

*How:* Eat a well-balanced diet, exercise regularly, and take your medications exactly as directed.

- **Regular exercise:**

Why? The benefits of regular exercise include improved circulation, pain relief, and general well-being.

*How:* Incorporate low-impact workouts like walking, swimming, and cycling. Before

beginning any new fitness programme,
consult with a healthcare physician.

- ***Benefits of a Healthy Diet:***

*Why?* A balanced diet contains key nutrients
that promote nerve health.
*How*: Eat a mix of fruits and vegetables,
whole grains, lean proteins, and healthy fats.
Consider contacting a dietitian for
personalised advice.

- ***Maintain a Healthy Weight:***

*Why?* Excess weight can worsen neuropathy
symptoms, especially in feet.
How: To reach and maintain a healthy
weight, eat a well-balanced diet and exercise
regularly.

- ***Quit Smoking:***

*Why?* Smoking can reduce blood flow and
worsen neuropathy symptoms.
*How:* Seek help from smoking cessation
programmes, pharmaceuticals, or
counselling.

- ***Limit Alcohol Consumption:***

*Why?* Excessive alcohol intake might cause nerve damage.

*How:* If you drink alcohol, do it in moderation and according to your healthcare provider's instructions.

- ***Manage Stress:***

*Why?* Stress can worsen neuropathy symptoms.

*How:* Incorporate stress-management strategies like meditation, deep breathing, yoga, or mindfulness into your daily routine.

- ***Foot Care:***

*Why?* Proper foot care is crucial for neuropathy patients, especially those with diabetes.

*How:* Check your feet for wounds or sores on a regular basis, wear comfortable and supportive shoes, and maintain proper foot cleanliness.

- ***Adequate Sleep:***

*Why:* Quality sleep promotes overall health and can alleviate neuropathy symptoms.
*How*: Establish a consistent sleep schedule, develop a pleasant sleeping environment, and address any sleep issues.

- ***Medication Management:***

*Why?* Taking prescribed drugs can help reduce symptoms and prevent progression.
*How:* Follow your healthcare provider's instructions for taking drugs and quickly express any adverse effects or concerns.

- ***Regular Medical Check-Ups:***

*Why?* Regular monitoring of general health allows possible concerns to be identified and addressed as soon a possible.
*How*: Attend planned medical appointments, follow up with experts, and express any changes in symptoms.

- ***Warm Baths or Massages***:

*Why?* These treatments may help alleviate neuropathy symptoms.

*How:* Take baths with warm (not hot) water and try light massages to increase circulation and relieve soreness.

It is critical to work with a healthcare expert to create a thorough strategy that is suited to your unique condition and needs. Individual cases of neuropathy differ, and personalised treatment offers the most effective management options.

# CHAPTER 9: 10 DAY MEAL PLAN



***Breakfast:***

Nutrient-packed smoothie with berries, spinach, almond milk, and a scoop of protein powder.

***Lunch:***

Grilled chicken breast salad with mixed greens, cherry tomatoes, cucumber, and a lemon-tahini dressing.

***Dinner:***

Baked salmon with quinoa and steamed broccoli.

Day 2:

***Breakfast:***

Whole grain toast with avocado and poached eggs.

***Lunch:***

Lentil soup with a side of mixed greens.

***Dinner:***

Stir-fried tofu with colourful bell peppers and brown rice.

## Day 3:

***Breakfast:***

Greek yogurt parfait with mixed berries, chia seeds, and a drizzle of honey.

***Lunch:***

Turkey and vegetable wrap with whole grain tortilla.

***Dinner:***

Shrimp and vegetable skewers with quinoa.

## Day 4:

***Breakfast:***

Oatmeal topped with sliced bananas, walnuts, and a sprinkle of cinnamon.

***Lunch:***

Quinoa salad with chickpeas, cherry tomatoes, cucumber, and feta cheese.

**Dinner:**

Grilled chicken with sweet potato wedges and sautéed spinach.

## Day 5:

**Breakfast:**

Avocado and spinach omelette with whole grain toast.

**Lunch:**

Tuna salad with mixed greens, cherry tomatoes, olives, and a light vinaigrette.

**Dinner:**

Baked cod with asparagus and quinoa.

## Day 6:

**Breakfast:**

Nut and seed smoothie with almond milk, flaxseeds, and a handful of mixed berries.

**Lunch:**

Whole grain wrap with hummus, sliced cucumber, shredded carrots, and turkey.

***Dinner:***

Vegetable stir-fry with tofu and brown rice.

## Day 7:

***Breakfast:***

Whole grain pancakes topped with fresh berries and a dollop of Greek yogurt.

***Lunch:***

Quinoa and black bean bowl with avocado, salsa, and lime.

***Dinner:***

Baked chicken breast with roasted Brussels sprouts and quinoa.

## Day 8:

***Breakfast:***

Greek yogurt smoothie with mango, banana, and a handful of spinach.

***Lunch:***

Salmon and vegetable salad with a lemon-olive oil dressing.

*Dinner:*

Lentil and vegetable curry with brown rice.

## Day 9:

*Breakfast:*

Chia seed pudding with almond milk and topped with sliced strawberries.

*Lunch:*

Turkey and vegetable stir-fry with quinoa.

*Dinner:*

Grilled shrimp skewers with a side of roasted sweet potatoes.

## Day 10:

*Breakfast:*

Whole grain toast with almond butter and sliced bananas.

*Lunch:*

Spinach and feta omelette with a side of
mixed berries.

### Dinner:

Baked cod with a side of quinoa and steamed
broccoli.

# CHAPTER 10:
# CONCLUSION

In summary, a neuropathy diet cookbook for beginners provides a straightforward and practical guide to selecting healthier food choices that may benefit nerve health. Individuals may produce delightful meals while improving their overall health by concentrating on nutrient-dense, whole foods and combining a range of flavours and textures. The cookbook emphasises the necessity of keeping blood sugar constant, eating lean proteins, and getting lots of fruits and vegetables.

The recipes presented are intended to be simple for beginners, allowing them to experiment with a neuropathy-friendly diet without feeling overwhelmed. The incorporation of nutrient-dense smoothies, lean proteins, whole grains, and fibre-rich meals gives a comprehensive approach to meeting the demands of neuropathy patients. Furthermore, the emphasis on thoughtful replacements, portion management, and altering classic recipes guarantees that people may eat delicious food while sticking to nutritional guidelines.

Finally, the neuropathy diet cookbook is a helpful resource for persons dealing with neuropathy, providing a practical and feasible approach to maintaining a balanced and nutritious diet for better overall health.

**STAY HEALTHY!**

MEAL
PLANNER

*D*AILY

DATE

BREAKFAST

NOTES

LUNCH

SNACK

ITEMS LIST

DINNER

# MEAL PLANNER

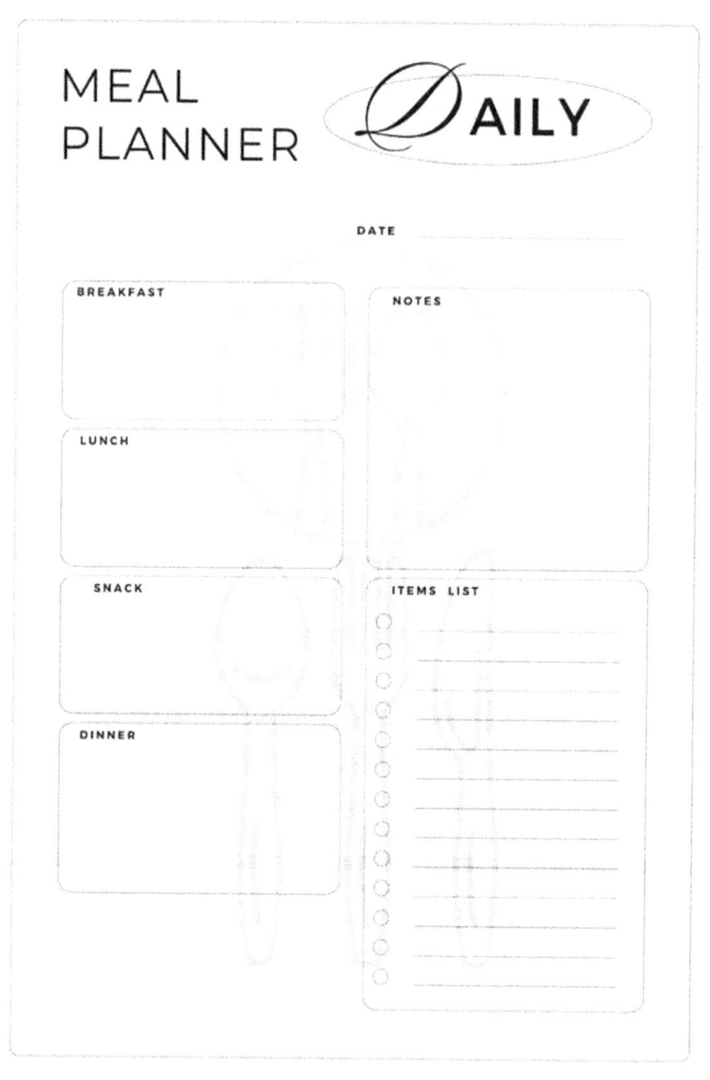

**DAILY**

DATE

BREAKFAST

LUNCH

SNACK

DINNER

NOTES

ITEMS LIST

# MEAL PLANNER

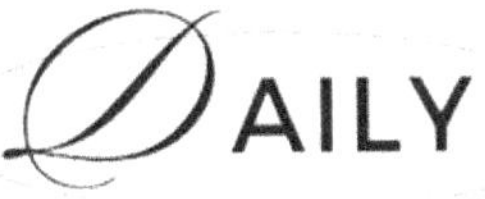

AILY

DATE

BREAKFAST

NOTES

LUNCH

SNACK

ITEMS LIST

DINNER

# MEAL PLANNER

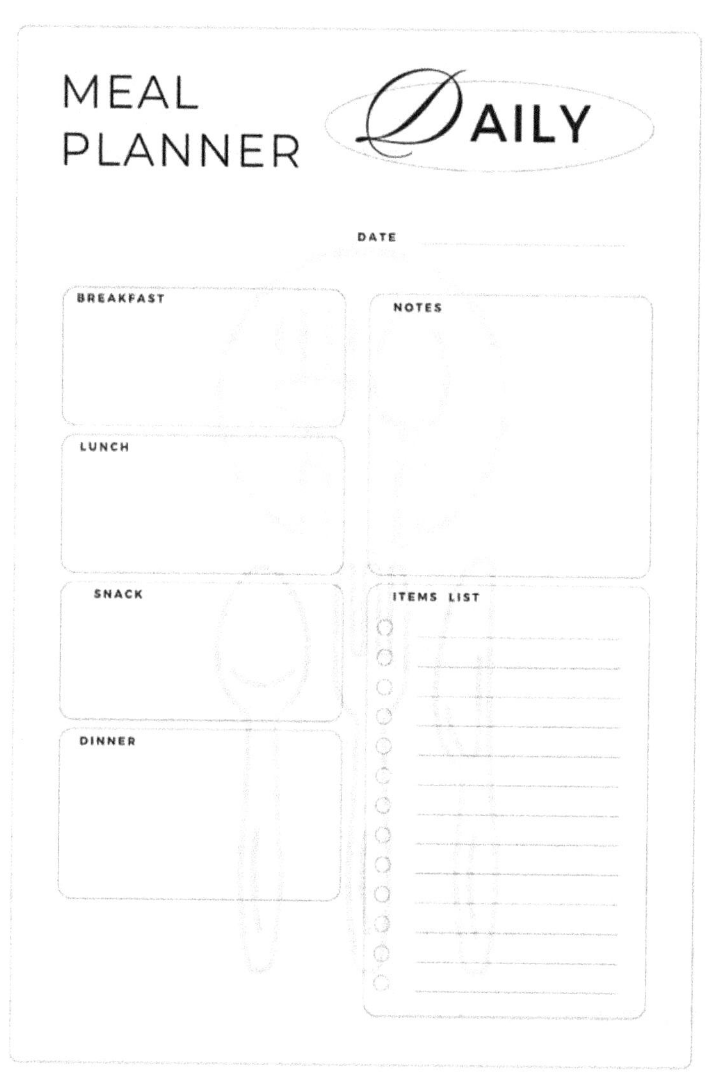

**DAILY**

DATE

BREAKFAST

LUNCH

SNACK

DINNER

NOTES

ITEMS LIST

# MEAL PLANNER

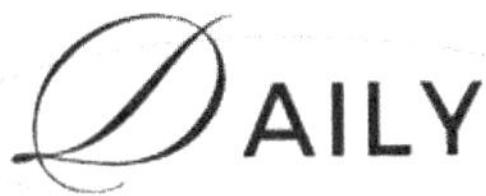

DATE

BREAKFAST

NOTES

LUNCH

SNACK

ITEMS LIST

DINNER

# MEAL PLANNER

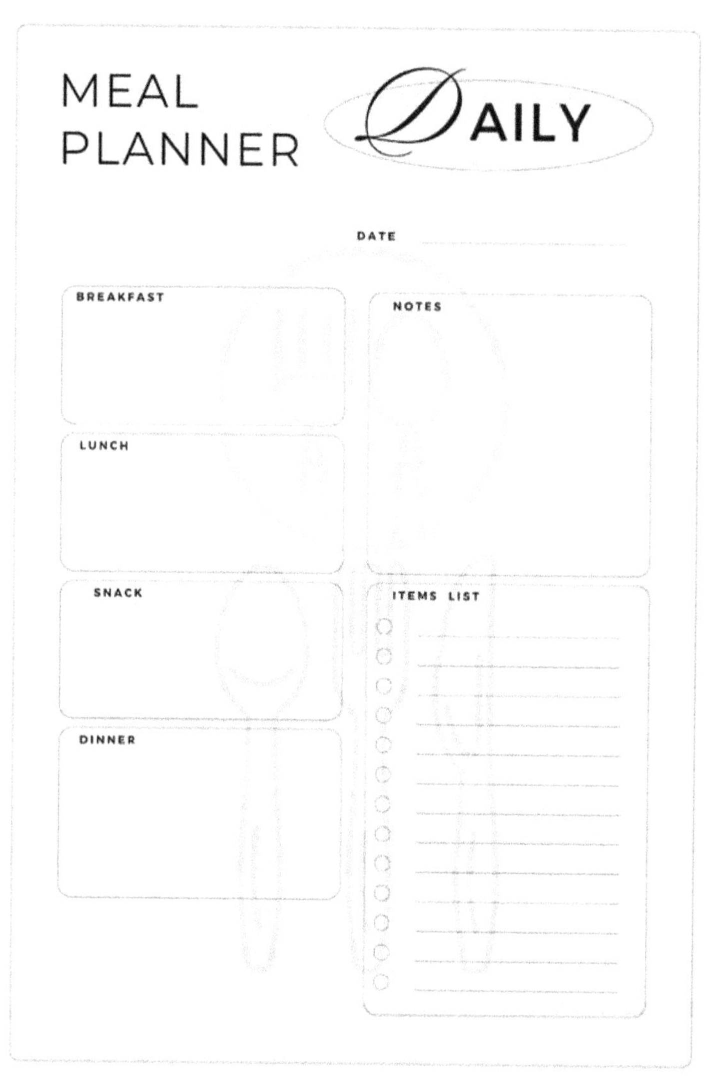

DAILY

DATE

BREAKFAST

LUNCH

SNACK

DINNER

NOTES

ITEMS LIST

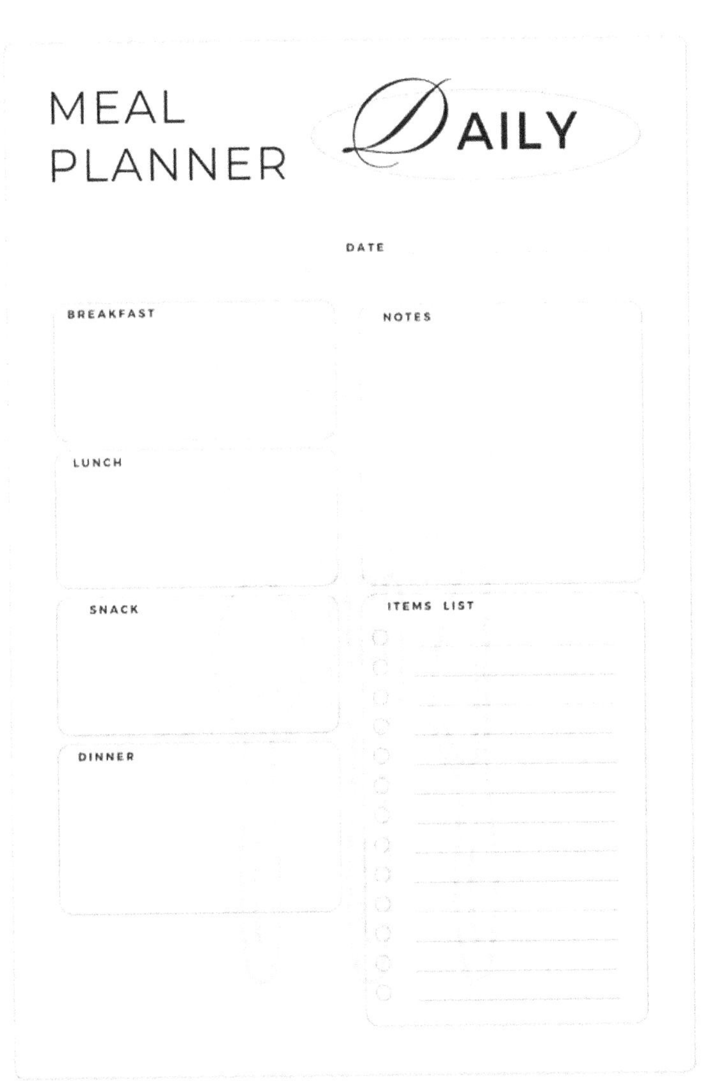
MEAL
PLANNER
DAILY
DATE
BREAKFAST
NOTES
LUNCH
SNACK
ITEMS LIST
DINNER

# MEAL PLANNER

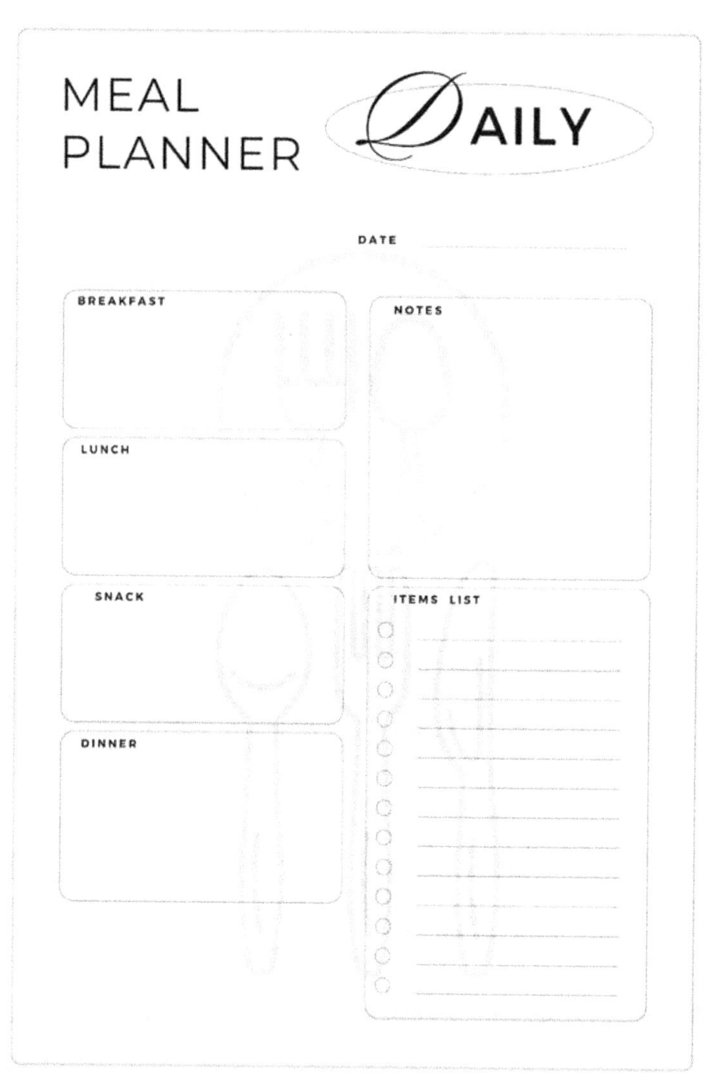

**DAILY**

DATE

**BREAKFAST**

**LUNCH**

**SNACK**

**DINNER**

**NOTES**

**ITEMS LIST**

# MEAL PLANNER

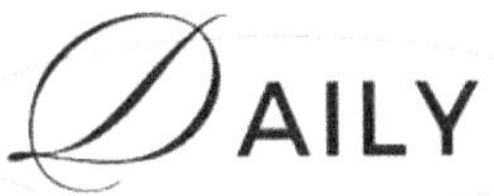

DATE

BREAKFAST

NOTES

LUNCH

SNACK

ITEMS LIST

DINNER

# MEAL PLANNER

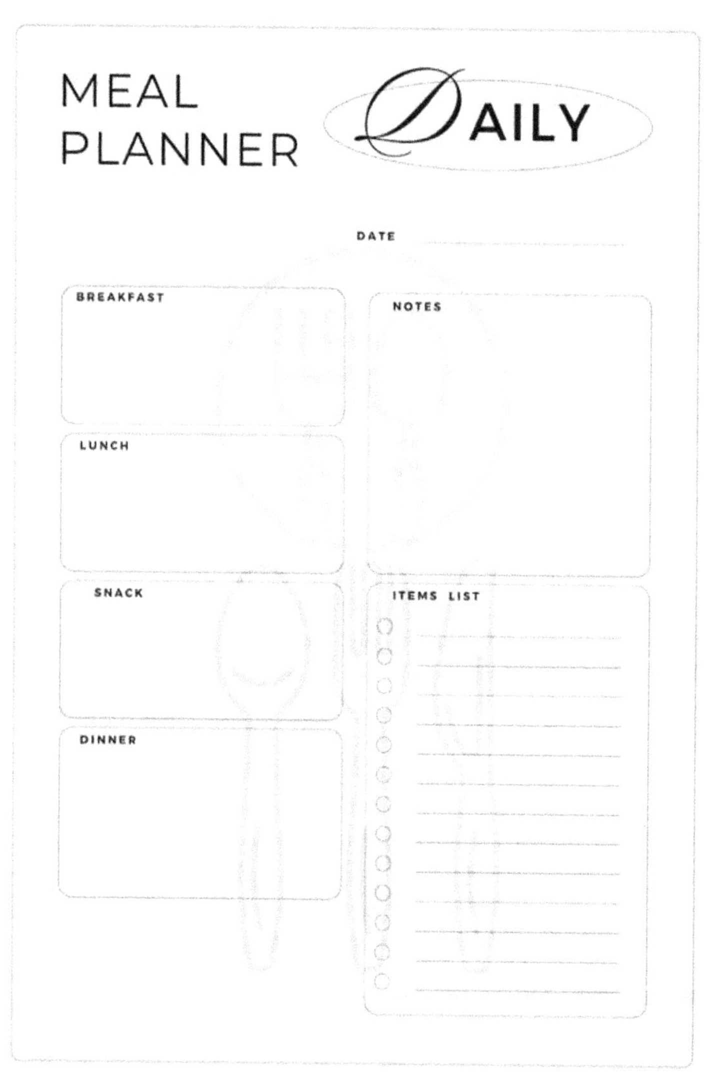

DAILY

DATE

**BREAKFAST**

**LUNCH**

**SNACK**

**DINNER**

**NOTES**

**ITEMS LIST**